MENINGITIS NUTRITION FOR BEGINNERS

Optimizing Health And Healing Through Targeted Dietary Strategies And Nutritional Insights For Meningitis Recovery

DR. JACE ZAYDEN

Table of Contents

DISCLAIMER

The information provided in the book is intended for general informational purposes only. The content of this book should not be considered a substitute for professional medical advice, diagnosis, or treatment.

Readers are advised to consult with a qualified healthcare professional for medical advice tailored to their individual circumstances.

The author has made every effort to ensure that the information in this book is accurate and up-to-date at the time of publication. However, medical knowledge is constantly evolving, and new research may emerge that could impact the information presented. The author disclaims any responsibility for any adverse effects or consequences resulting from the use of the information provided in this book.

References or mentions of individuals, products, websites, organizations, or other names within this book are for informational purposes only and do not constitute an endorsement. The author has no affiliations with, and makes no endorsements of, any third-party entities mentioned. Readers are encouraged to conduct their own research and exercise their judgment when considering any external resources or recommendations.

The author and the publisher shall have neither liability nor responsibility to any person or entity with respect to any loss, damage, or injury caused or alleged to be caused directly or indirectly by the information contained in this book. Any reliance on the information within this book is at the reader's own risk.

By reading this book, the reader acknowledges and agrees to the terms of this disclaimer. If the reader does not agree with these terms, they should not use the information provided in this book.

ABOUT THIS BOOK

This book entitled "Meningitis Nutrition" is a seminal work in the field of healthcare literature, as it addresses a frequently neglected but crucial aspect of patient treatment. The introductory sections of this book establish the context by presenting an all-encompassing synopsis of meningitis, elucidating its intricacies and the profound consequences it imposes on individuals. Exploring the core issues at hand, the chapters devoted to nutritional considerations are of immense value, as they underscore the critical significance of adequate nutrition in the process of recuperating from meningitis.

This book provides a comprehensive analysis of the significance of nutrition in the process of recovering from meningitis. It emphasizes the direct relationship that a balanced diet has with improved outcomes of recovery. The text effectively addresses the nutritional obstacles that are intrinsic to cases of meningitis and provides practical advice on dietary recommendations that are optimized for recovery. The importance of fluid ingestion and hydration is underscored, as they are recognized to be crucial components in the process of recovery.

This book contains an abundance of information about nutrient-dense foods that are particularly advantageous for individuals recovering from meningitis. Additionally, it delves into an examination of the vital vitamins and minerals that are indispensable for achieving optimal nutrition throughout this period. The comprehensive listing of special dietary considerations in the book demonstrates its earnestness in attending to the varied requirements of patients.

An aspect that sets this book apart is its pragmatic methodology, which offers recommendations for monitoring and modifying nutrition strategies in response to the ever-changing nature of recovery. Furthermore, it urges cooperation with healthcare practitioners and emphasizes the value of a multidisciplinary strategy in providing treatment for patients.

This book's practicality is increased by the incorporation of case studies, which provide tangible examples of the difficulties and achievements associated with the implementation of nutritional strategies in cases of meningitis. The chapter about nutritional support for long-term effects expands the applicability of this book beyond immediate recuperation, discussing the lasting consequences of meningitis on individuals.

In conclusion, this book astutely explores preventive nutrition strategies, acknowledging the criticality of proactive measures in preventing the initiation or reappearance of meningitis. Fundamentally, "Meningitis Nutrition" serves as an essential manual, bridging the crucial chasm that exists between nutritional support and medical treatment. It provides healthcare professionals, caregivers, and patients equally with an authoritative reference.

CHAPTER ONE

NUTRITION FOR MENINGITIS: SUSTAINING THE BODY AND MIND THROUGHOUT RECOVERY

Introduction

Meningitis is an inflammation of the membranes encircling the brain and spinal cord that has the potential to be fatal. Diverse infectious agents, including bacteria, viruses, fungi, and parasites, are capable of causing it. Prompt medical attention is required due to the severe nature of meningitis; however, it is frequently treated with hospitalization and medication. Nevertheless, medical intervention is not the sole determinant of recovery; adequate nutrition is vital in bolstering the body's innate healing mechanisms and promoting a more complete recuperation for those afflicted with meningitis.

A Synopsis Of Meningitis

The rapid initiation and potential for severe complications of meningitis render it a substantial public health issue. A variety of symptoms may result from inflammation of the meninges, which are the protective membranes that envelop the brain and spinal cord. These may include fever, headache, rigidity in the neck, and sensitivity to light. Although less prevalent than viral meningitis, bacterial meningitis is more severe and, if not treated promptly, can lead to long-term complications or even mortality.

In most cases, meningitis is managed with the administration of antibiotics or antiviral drugs, contingent upon the etiological agent. Additionally vital are supportive care components like pain management and intravenous fluids. Hospitalization may be required during the acute phase of meningitis; however, the recuperation process transcends the preliminary medical intervention.

Throughout the rehabilitation period, nutrition is crucial for bolstering the immune system, resupplying energy stores, and promoting general health.

Considerations Regarding Nutrition In Meningitis

The provision of nutritional support is critical for the recuperation of individuals afflicted with meningitis. Amidst the acute phase, during which individuals may manifest symptoms such as diminished appetite or dysphagia, it is critical to furnish them with foods that are readily digestible and rich in nutrients. In extreme circumstances, intravenous nutrition may be required to ensure that the body receives essential nutrients despite the restriction of oral consumption.

Maintaining sufficient hydration is of utmost importance to avert complications and facilitate the recovery process. Illness-related fever and increased metabolic demands can result in dehydration; therefore, regular fluid consumption is crucial. Regular hydration is crucial for the maintenance of electrolyte balance, which is essential for many physiological processes such as nerve conduction and muscle contraction.

Protein is an essential component in the process of healing, as it performs vital functions in tissue repair and immune system support. People recovering from meningitis may experience muscle atrophy or frailty; therefore, protein consumption is crucial for the re-establishment and maintenance of muscle mass. Lean meats, poultry, fish, eggs, dairy products, legumes, and plant-based alternatives are all excellent sources of protein.

Selenium, vitamin C, vitamin D, and zinc are examples of minerals and vitamins that support the immune system and overall health. Providing the body with sufficient quantities of these nutrients can aid in the fight against infections and promote recovery. Nuts, fruits, vegetables, and whole cereals contain an abundance of vital vitamins and minerals.

Omega-3 fatty acids, which are present in walnuts, rich salmon, and flaxseeds, have the potential to support neurological health and reduce inflammation in the brain due to their anti-inflammatory properties. The incorporation of these dietary sources of healthful lipids may enhance the general welfare of individuals undergoing recovery from meningitis.

Significance Of Nutrition In The Recovery From Meningitis

The significance of nutrition in the rehabilitation of meningitis cannot be emphasized enough. A nutrient-dense and nutritionally balanced diet is crucial for several reasons:

1. Immune Function Support: Meningitis imposes a substantial burden on the immune system. Adequate nutrition supplies the essential components for immune cells, thereby bolstering the body's capacity to combat pathogens and facilitating expedited recuperation.

2. Restoring Energy Stores: The amount of energy expended while unwell can be substantial. Sufficient caloric consumption guarantees that the body possesses sufficient energy to sustain vital functions, thereby averting fatigue and facilitating the overall process of recuperation.

3. Preventing Complications: Muscle atrophy, cognitive impairments, and frailty are all potential complications that may result from meningitis. Adequate protein consumption, in particular, aids in the prevention of these complications through its positive impact on cognitive function and muscle repair.

4. Preserving Hydration: Dehydration is a prevalent issue that can worsen symptoms and impede the recuperation process when experienced during an illness. Ensuring adequate hydration is critical for optimal physiological functioning and facilitates the elimination of contaminants from the body.

5. Supporting Neurological Health: Antioxidants and omega-3 fatty acids are nutrients that promote neurological health. Incorporating these foods into one's diet may facilitate cognitive function support and inflammation reduction in the brain during recovery from meningitis.

In conclusion, a holistic approach to meningitis recovery must incorporate nutrition as a crucial component. In addition to medical interventions, nutrient supplementation promotes optimal body healing and reduces the likelihood of complications. Healthcare professionals, such as nutritionists and dietitians, are of paramount importance in the formulation of personalized nutrition strategies that address the unique requirements of individuals with meningitis. This facilitates a more expeditious and resilient recuperation.

Nutritional Difficulties Encountered In Meningitis

Patients afflicted with meningitis, an inflammation of the membranes encompassing the brain and spinal cord, may encounter considerable nutritional obstacles. Individuals may experience impaired nutrient absorption and digestion due to the severity of the illness and its accompanying symptoms. Meningitis is characterized by nutritional challenges that are influenced by a variety of factors; therefore, dietary considerations must be incorporated into the overall treatment strategy.

A significant obstacle encountered by individuals afflicted with meningitis is the frequent occurrence of appetite loss. Symptoms of the infection and inflammation include vertigo, vomiting, and an overall aversion to food. Consequently, individuals may have difficulty obtaining the nutrients they require, which could potentially result in weight loss and compromised immune function.

In addition, metabolic demands increase when the body is afflicted with a disease such as encephalitis. Supplementary nutrients and energy are necessary for the immune system to combat the infection and promote recovery. The increased need for nutrients may cause the body to exhaust its reserves, underscoring the criticality of consuming sufficient nutrients while recovering.

An additional element that contributes to nutritional difficulties is the potential repercussions of meningitis treatments. Certain medications have the potential to disrupt appetite, digestion, and nutrient assimilation, thereby compounding the challenges that patients are already confronted with in getting enough nutrition.

To confront these obstacles, medical professionals must diligently oversee and regulate the nutritional status of patients afflicted with meningitis. This may entail the implementation of dietary adjustments, the utilization of nutritional supplements, and vigilant surveillance of weight and nutritional indicators. Medical professionals, dietitians, and caregivers must work in concert to ensure that patients receive the essential nutrients required for their recovery.

CHAPTER TWO

Advised Dietary Principles

It is imperative to establish unambiguous dietary protocols for individuals undergoing recovery from meningitis. The purpose of these dietary recommendations is to supply the essential nutrients required for immune system support, wound healing, and the prevention of malnutrition-related complications. Although individual dietary requirements may differ, the nutritional management of patients with meningitis can be guided by certain general recommendations.

1. A sufficient caloric intake is crucial to satisfy the heightened energy requirements that occur during periods of illness. Prioritizing nutrient-dense foods is crucial for ensuring that the body is supplied with calories and vital vitamins and minerals. Individuals with a diminished appetite may benefit from consuming meals on a smaller scale and more frequently.

2. Protein is an essential nutrient for immune function and tissue repair. Consuming lean meats, poultry, fish, dairy products, legumes, and seeds, among other nutritious protein sources, can aid in the recovery process.

3. Maintaining adequate hydration is critical, particularly in the presence of fever and vomiting. Encourage the consumption of clear fluids, electrolyte-rich beverages, and oral rehydration solutions if necessary. It is critical to monitor fluid homeostasis to avert dehydration.

4. Vitamins and Minerals: An optimal consumption of vitamins and minerals is ensured by a balanced diet that is abundant in fruits and vegetables. Selenium and zinc, in addition to vitamins A, C, and E, are particularly important for immune function and may facilitate recovery.

5. Constipation is a frequent complication of medication use and illness. By incorporating foods that are high in fiber, such as whole cereals, fruits, and vegetables, this issue can be mitigated.

Tailored dietary regimens may be required, taking into account the particular symptoms, dietary inclinations, and preexisting medical conditions of the patient. Consistent monitoring and necessary modifications to the dietary regimen are imperative as the individual advances through the phases of recuperation.

Intake Of Fluids And Hydration

It is essential to maintain a healthy fluid balance when treating meningitis, as dehydration can worsen symptoms and impede recovery. Fluid loss can be induced by fever, perspiration, regurgitation, and an elevated respiratory rate; therefore, it is critical to emphasize the importance of maintaining adequate hydration.

It is imperative to motivate individuals diagnosed with meningitis to consume ample fluids, such as electrolyte-rich beverages, water, and oral rehydration solutions when necessary. Preventing dehydration and preserving electrolyte balance are the objectives.

It is critical to closely monitor urinary output, dehydration, and overall hydration status, particularly in critical situations that may require intravenous fluid administration.

When individuals are unable to adequately ingest fluids through oral means, medical professionals may opt to administer hydration via intravenous means. This allows for the immediate and regulated administration of fluids and electrolytes to sustain the physiological requirements of the body.

Notably, alcohol and caffeine have the potential to cause dehydration and should be consumed in moderation. To promote optimal hydration, greater emphasis should be placed on non-caffeinated and non-alcoholic beverages.

Caregivers fulfill a vital function in overseeing and promoting fluid consumption, given that patients afflicted with meningitis may experience hunger and thirst as a result of additional symptoms including vertigo. Consistent communication with healthcare providers regarding adjustments in fluid consumption or indications of dehydration is critical to facilitate prompt interventions.

Foods Rich In Nutrients For Meningitis Patients

It is of the utmost importance that individuals rehabilitating from meningitis consume nutrient-dense foods, as these contain vitamins, minerals, and other vital nutrients that are required for immune support and healing. A diverse selection of nutrient-dense foods can be utilized to meet particular nutritional requirements while recovering.

1. Consume fruits and vegetables; they are abundant in immune-supporting antioxidants and vitamins A, C, and E. The diet should consist of vibrant vegetables, berries, citrus fruits, and verdant plants.

2. Excellent sources of protein include lean meats, poultry, fish, eggs, dairy products, legumes, and seeds. Protein is essential for immune function, tissue repair, and overall recovery.

3. Whole grains, including quinoa, brown rice, oatmeal, and whole wheat, are rich in essential nutrients and fiber. They promote digestive health and aid in the prevention of constipation.

4. Dairy products and plant-based alternatives that have been fortified with calcium and vitamin D are essential for maintaining healthy bones and promoting overall well-being.

5. Healthy lipids, including those found in avocado, almonds, seeds, and olive oil, aid in the absorption of fat-soluble vitamins and provide energy support.

6. Foods that are rich in water: Soups, watermelon, and cucumber are examples of hydrating foods that can aid in overall fluid consumption and hydration.

Cultural sensitivity, personal preferences, and dietary restrictions should all be incorporated into meal planning. Collaborating with a healthcare professional or dietitian guarantees that dietary suggestions are to the unique requirements of the individual and facilitate their recuperation from meningitis.

For individuals recovering from meningitis, addressing nutritional challenges, adhering to recommended dietary guidelines, emphasizing adequate fluid intake, and incorporating nutrient-dense foods are, in summary, essential components of comprehensive care. Healthcare professionals, patients, and caregivers must adopt a collaborative approach to customize dietary strategies to suit individual requirements and facilitate optimal recovery.

Minerals And Vitamins In The Nutrition For Meningitis

Meningitis is a critical medical condition distinguished by the inflammatory reaction of the membranes that protect the brain and spinal cord. Although medical intervention is of utmost importance in the treatment of meningitis, adequate nutrition significantly contributes to immune system support and facilitates the process of recuperation. Vitamins and minerals are fundamental constituents of meningitis nutrition, enhancing the body's capacity to combat infections and contributing to overall health.

Vitamin C is an essential vitamin in encephalitis nutrition. Vitamin C, which is recognized for its immune-enhancing attributes, facilitates the synthesis of collagen, a vital protein in the process of wound repair. In the context of meningitis, when the immune system is significantly taxed, it is vital to maintain optimal vitamin C levels. Incorporating vitamin C-rich foods into one's diet, including citrus fruits, strawberries, and bell peppers, can be beneficial for promoting recovery.

Vitamin D is also an essential component in the realm of meningitis nutrition. This vitamin possesses anti-inflammatory properties and is vital for immune system function. Although sunlight is an inherent source of vitamin D, individuals afflicted with meningitis should supplement their intake with dietary sources such as fatty salmon, fortified dairy products, and egg yolks. Sufficient levels of vitamin D have the potential to expedite the recuperation process and mitigate the likelihood of complications.

Essential for immune system functionality, minerals such as selenium and zinc can facilitate the recovery process. Zinc, which is abundant in nuts, cereals, and meat, is essential for immune cell function and wound healing. Selenium, which is found in whole grains, fish, and Brazil nuts, functions as an antioxidant and bolsters the immune system's ability to combat infections. Consuming these minerals is essential for those who are in the process of recuperating from meningitis.

Brain health is dependent on B vitamins, specifically B6, B9 (folate), and B12. B12 in particular may contribute to the recovery from meningitis. The maintenance of nerve cells and the synthesis of neurotransmitters are processes facilitated by these vitamins. Fortified cereals, poultry, fish, and leafy vegetables are excellent sources of B vitamins and should be incorporated into the diet to aid in the rehabilitation of meningitis by supporting neurological function.

In conclusion, for meningitis nutrition, a well-balanced diet abundant in vitamins C and D, zinc, selenium, and B vitamins is essential. These essential nutrients promote overall health, facilitate wound healing, and fortify the immune system, thereby assisting individuals in their more efficient recovery from this critical ailment.

CHAPTER THREE

Dietary Special Considerations

The management of meningitis necessitates dietary modifications in addition to medical interventions to promote recovery and reduce the risk of complications. Particular dietary considerations are crucial in meningitis nutrition to meet the distinct requirements of those afflicted with this severe infection.

Hydration maintenance is among the foremost factors to be mindful of. Dehydration may result from meningitis, particularly when marked by fever and vomiting. It is essential to consume sufficient fluids to prevent dehydration and aid in the body's recovery. For proper hydration, water, electrolyte-rich beverages, and clear broths are suggested.

When an individual has meningitis, it is critical to adhere to a diet that is rich in essential nutrients. Sufficient caloric intake from a well-balanced diet is critical for the overall recovery process, as the body's energy demands increase during illness. Prioritize the consumption of nutrient-dense foods, such as lean proteins, whole cereals, fruits, and vegetables, to obtain vital vitamins and minerals.

Meningitis can cause diminished appetite and difficulty ingesting in certain affected individuals. It may be necessary to modify the diet to incorporate milder or pureed foods in such circumstances. Soups, smoothies, and mashed vegetables can provide vital nutrients while avoiding an undue burden on the digestive system.

Food safety should also be taken into account, given that meningitis has the potential to compromise the immune system. To prevent secondary infections, it is vital to avoid consuming fresh or undercooked foods and to observe appropriate food hygiene.

Nausea is a frequently encountered symptom of meningitis observed in affected individuals. It may be beneficial to consume smaller, more frequent meals to manage this. Additionally, improving overall food tolerance and reducing vertigo may be accomplished by avoiding fatty and spicy foods.

It is crucial to acknowledge that dietary requirements can differ among individuals; therefore, it is essential to seek guidance from healthcare professionals, such as registered dietitians. By the individual's nutritional status, underlying conditions, and the severity of the malady, they are capable of generating individualized dietary recommendations.

In summary, when it comes to meningitis nutrition, specific dietary considerations encompass hydration, nutrient density, texture adjustments, food safety, and symptom control. In conjunction with healthcare professionals, a customized nutritional regimen is essential for promoting recovery and averting complications related to meningitis.

Observing And Modifying Dietary Plans

Monitoring and modifying nutrition plans are essential components of meningitis management, as they guarantee that patients receive the essential nutrients required for recovery and address any emergent complications or alterations in health conditions.

Consistent monitoring of nutritional consumption entails evaluating the dietary patterns of the individual, encompassing the quantities and varieties of foods ingested. This method facilitates the detection of deficiencies or excesses in particular nutrients and permits the implementation of modifications to optimize nutrition. Healthcare practitioners, with registered dietitians in particular, have a critical responsibility in overseeing nutrition plans and implementing any required adjustments.

Nutritional assessments may encompass activities such as monitoring fluctuations in body weight, analyzing dietary inclinations, and assessing concentrations of vital nutrients in the bloodstream. For instance, the utilization of blood tests to monitor vitamin and mineral levels can facilitate the detection of deficiencies that might necessitate supplementation.

Another critical element to consider when monitoring nutrition in cases of meningitis is fluid balance. Dehydration can potentially affect individuals who experience fever, vomiting, or a reduction in fluid consumption.

Consistent monitoring of hydration levels and necessary modifications to fluid consumption is imperative to avert complications that may arise from dehydration.

Modifications to the dietary regimen might be necessary as the individual advances during the treatment phase. This is especially crucial in situations involving alterations in appetite, complications with digestion, or the emergence of additional symptoms. For example, in the case of dysphagia, it may be imperative to alter the consistency of foods or select alternative options that are abundant in nutrients.

Tailored nutrition strategies are imperative, given the wide range of requirements and reactions to meningitis. In addition, modifications may be necessary in consideration of the existence of pre-existing medical conditions or the utilization of particular medications that may influence nutritional needs.

It is vital for long-term health to educate individuals and their caregivers about nutrition during and after meningitis. This includes promoting healthy eating practices, disseminating information regarding the importance of maintaining a balanced diet, and ensuring sufficient intake of vital nutrients to facilitate continuous recovery.

In summary, the dynamic processes of monitoring and modifying nutrition programs are integral components of meningitis management. Consistent evaluations, personalized methodologies, and cooperation between healthcare practitioners and patients are critical for maximizing nutritional assistance, facilitating recuperation, and averting complications linked to insufficient nourishment.

Physical And Mental Nourishment

Meningitis, an inflammation of the meningeal and spinal cord-peripheral membranes, presents a substantial global health risk. Although medical interventions are of paramount importance in the treatment of meningitis, nutrition is frequently disregarded despite being a vital component of the recuperation process. This article explores multiple aspects of meningitis nutrition, including case studies, preventive nutrition strategies, nutritional support for long-term effects, and collaboration with healthcare professionals.

CHAPTER FOUR

Developing Partnerships With Healthcare Professionals: An Interdisciplinary Strategy

Collaboration with healthcare professionals is crucial for the successful management of nutrition associated with meningitis. Nutritionists, dietitians, physicians, and nurses must collaborate to customize dietary regimens that address the specific requirements of individuals with meningitis. Nutrient needs are influenced by the specific causative agent, the severity of meningitis, and the patient's overall health condition.

When engaging in collaborative efforts, it is crucial to address the obstacles that arise during the acute phase of meningitis. Throughout this phase, individuals might encounter symptoms such as reduced appetite, dysphagia, and modified gustatory perception. When oral intake is inadequate, nutritional interventions, including enteral and parenteral nutrition, are taken into account through a collaborative effort. Additionally, fluid and electrolyte balance must be closely monitored, particularly when meningitis causes increased fluid loss due to fever and perspiration.

In addition, healthcare practitioners must give precedence to ensuring that patients receive sufficient quantities of protein, vitamins, and minerals to bolster the immune system and facilitate the regeneration of bodily tissues. An optimal nutritional composition, comprising lean proteins, whole cereals, fruits, and vegetables, may facilitate an accelerated recuperation.

Education of patients is a fundamental component of collaboration. Healthcare personnel ought to provide patients with the authority to make well-informed dietary decisions, placing significant emphasis on the transformational role of nutrition. Consistent monitoring and modifications to dietary regimens by the patient's advancements are fundamental elements of collaborative healthcare.

Nutritional Case Studies For Meningitis: Insights Derived From Practical Experiences

An analysis of case studies yields significant insights regarding the pragmatic implementation of nutrition in the management of meningitis. These studies provide insights into the various nutritional obstacles that patients encounter and propose approaches to mitigate them.

Let us contemplate a scenario in which an individual afflicted with bacterial meningitis undergoes substantial muscle atrophy and weight loss throughout the acute phase. The nutritional intervention consists of a protein-rich, high-calorie diet designed to aid in recovery and promote muscle preservation. This case underscores the importance of customized nutrition plans that take into account the nutritional status, comorbidities, and treatment regimen of the individual.

An additional case study could center on a pediatric patient who has contracted viral meningitis, with an emphasis on the criticality of nutritional interventions tailored to the patient's age. Physicians, dietitians, and caregivers must work together in this situation to ensure that the child receives sufficient nutrition for growth and development.

The case studies highlight the ever-changing nature of nutrition for meningitis, underscoring the importance of being flexible and adaptable in the management of dietary intake. Healthcare practitioners may utilize these practical experiences to enhance their nutritional strategies when dealing with cases of meningitis.

Nutrient-Based Long-Term Effects Support: Nurturing Beyond Recovery

Long-term consequences of meningitis can manifest in cognitive and physical functions. A sustained commitment to nutritional support is required to manage these effects and promote overall health.

Personalized nutritional interventions may promote nerve regeneration and cognitive function in patients who have developed neurological complications after meningitis. Certain nutritional components, including omega-3 fatty acids, antioxidants, and particular vitamins, might contribute to the maintenance of optimal brain function. Involving neurologists and nutritionists in collaborative care is crucial to formulating comprehensive strategies that effectively target long-term neurological consequences.

Nutrition is once again an essential component in physical rehabilitation. Fatigue, joint pain, and muscle weakness are frequent complications of meningitis. In conjunction with targeted supplementation, adequate protein consumption can promote muscle strength and facilitate the restoration of physical function. The integration of physiotherapists and rehabilitation specialists into the collaborative effort guarantees a comprehensive strategy for providing sustained nutritional assistance.

Furthermore, it is crucial to incorporate mental health factors when providing nutritional support to individuals who are experiencing the enduring consequences of meningitis. Cognitive fatigue, anxiety, and depression can all affect dietary patterns. A collaborative approach involving psychiatrists, psychologists, and dietitians can be of assistance in addressing the psychological and emotional aspects of nutrition in such situations.

Strategies For Preventive Nutrition: Enhancing Immunity And Mitigating Potential Hazards

It is vital to implement preventive nutrition strategies to lower the risk of meningitis and promote overall health. Although vaccines play a crucial role in the prevention of specific strains of meningitis, a balanced diet also enhances the overall resilience of the immune system.

It is crucial to implement preventive measures by ensuring sufficient consumption of immune-boosting nutrients, including vitamin C, vitamin D, zinc, and antioxidants.

For community-wide health promotion, it is essential to collaborate with public health professionals to disseminate information regarding the role of nutrition in preventing infections, including meningitis.

Additionally, hydration is an essential component of preventive nutrition. Ensuring adequate fluid balance is vital for bolstering the body's defense mechanisms and mitigating the risk of infections. Healthcare professionals can effectively direct education campaigns that emphasize the criticality of adequate hydration as a preventive measure against meningitis and other contagious illnesses.

In summary, meningitis nutrition incorporates a wide range of factors, including preventive strategies, long-term support, and acute care collaboration. To nourish individuals afflicted with meningitis comprehensively and holistically, it is imperative to engage in effective collaboration with healthcare professionals, derive insights from case studies, consider long-term consequences, and adopt preventive nutrition strategies. By fostering interdisciplinary collaboration, it is possible to optimize nutritional interventions to augment recovery, mitigate complications, and advance overall well-being amidst this arduous condition.

Conclusion

In summary, nutrition is an essential component in the treatment and recuperation of those afflicted with meningitis. Adhering to a nutrient-dense and nutritionally balanced diet is imperative for bolstering the immune system, facilitating the recovery process, and averting complications that may arise from this potentially fatal condition.

In the acute phase of meningitis, when the body is experiencing significant physiological strain, it is critical to consume an adequate number of calories. Adequate nutrition plays a pivotal role in sustaining the body's increased energy requirements and bolstering its resistance against infection.

Vitamins C and E, zinc, and omega-3 fatty acids are essential nutrients due to their anti-inflammatory and antioxidant properties, which aid in the reduction of inflammation and promotion of overall recovery.

In addition, it is imperative to ensure adequate hydration to mitigate the risk of complications that may result from dehydration, which is a prevalent issue in the context of illness. Optimal recuperation is ensured by replenishing lost electrolytes and fluids, which assist in the restoration of normal bodily functions.

A critical consideration during the progression from the acute phase to recovery and rehabilitation is the consumption of nutrient-dense foods.

This consists of a variety of fruits, vegetables, lean proteins, and whole cereals that supply the body with the antioxidants, vitamins, and minerals it needs to repair and regain strength.

Fundamentally, a comprehensive and deliberate nutritional strategy constitutes an essential component of the holistic management of meningitis patients, fostering not only recuperation but also sustained health and overall welfare.

THE END